DEDICATION

This book is dedicated to all those who try to find long term solutions to their weight loss problems. It can be difficult but with dedication, a solution can be found.

TABLE OF CONTENTS

Intermittent Fasting: The Guide to the Fast Diet for Weight Loss

How to Make the Fast Diet or Intermittent Fasting Work

By: Stacie Williams

9781632874641

PUBLISHERS NOTES

Disclaimer – Speedy Publishing, LLC

This publication is intended to provide helpful and informative material. It is not intended to diagnose, treat, cure, or prevent any health problem or condition, nor is intended to replace the advice of a physician. No action should be taken solely on the contents of this book. Always consult your physician or qualified health-care professional on any matters regarding your health and before adopting any suggestions in this book or drawing inferences from it.

The author and publisher specifically disclaim all responsibility for any liability, loss or risk, personal or otherwise, which is incurred as a consequence, directly or indirectly, from the use or application of any contents of this book.

Any and all product names referenced within this book are the trademarks of their respective owners. None of these owners have sponsored, authorized, endorsed, or approved this book.

Always read all information provided by the manufacturers' product labels before using their products. The author and publisher are not responsible for claims made by manufacturers.

This book was originally printed before 2014. This is an adapted reprint by Speedy Publishing, LLC with newly updated content designed to help readers with much more accurate and timely information and data.

Speedy Publishing, LLC

40 E Main Street,

Newark

Delaware

19711

Contact Us: 1-888-248-4521

Website: http://www.speedypublishing.com

REPRINTED Paperback Edition: ISBN: 9781632874641

Manufactured in the United States of America

INTRODUCTION- FAT BURNING BASICS

If you're overweight, you are not a bad person. You're simply overweight. But it's important to lose the extra pounds so you'll look good, feel healthier and develop a sense of pride and self-esteem. Once you've lost the fat, you'll need to maintain your weight.

Most Americans pack on those extra pounds by eating the wrong things. Changing these poor eating habits is the key to long-term success. Knowledge – along with the right food – is the key.

When humans lived in caves, they didn't know anything about preserving and storing food. They spent all their waking time and energy hunting and gathering food. When they had it, they gobbled it down fast. Instead of storing food in pantries or cupboards, they stored energy in their bodies in the form of fat to burn during periods when there was little or nothing to eat.

Each year, it was absolutely vital for them to put on a good layer of fat during the warm spring and summer months. That was the only way they could guarantee their survival during the lean and mean winter months.

And since women bore the young, they needed more energy to sustain themselves and their babies, and that meant they were usually heavier.

Even though we no longer live in caves, we have inherited and maintained this basic mechanism for fat storage from our hunting and gathering ancestors.

Each one of us is born with a certain number of fat cells. How many of these fat cells you possess depend on genetics. If you have a lot of fat cells, maybe your ancestors were the biggest people in the tribe, which was a good thing because they had the best chances of survival.

You can never get rid of fat cells, but – unfortunately – you can add to them. Depending upon what you eat, your body will manufacture new far cells. And like those you were born with, they never go away.

That doesn't mean you're doomed to be fat once you put on extra pounds. It is possible to shrink fat cells. That's what happens when you lose weight. You burn up the fat stored in those big fat cells. Think of them as balloons. Burning off the fat inside them has the same effect as letting the air out of a balloon.

A good weight loss program requires a certain amount of intake restriction – the consumption of fewer calories. You burn off the fat by eating less fat and becoming more active.

To guarantee a lifetime of weight-control success, you have to change the type of foods you eat, so that you ingest less fat and still get the vitamins, minerals, trace elements, protein, fat and carbohydrates your body needs to thrive.

Extremely low-calorie diets may help you shed pounds quickly, but they'll lead to failure in the long run.

That's because humans are genetically protected against starvation. During food shortages, our bodies slow down our metabolisms and burn less energy so we can stay alive.

A part of our brain called the hypothalamus keeps us on an even weight keep by creating a "set point." That's the weight where we feel comfortable. The hypothalamus determines this point based on the level of consumption it's used to. It seeks to keep our weight constant, even if that point is over what it should be.

When we drastically cut back our food intake, the brain thinks the body is starving, and in an effort to preserve life, it slows the metabolism. Soon the pounds stop coming off. Consequently, we grow hungry and uncomfortable and then eat more. And then the diet fails.

How can you compensate for this metabolic slow-down? The answer is that you have to change the nutritional composition of the foods you eat. You will have to cut down on total calories — that's absolutely basic to weight loss. More important, however, is reducing the percentage of total calories you are getting from fat.

That's how you'll avoid starvation panic in your system. At the same time, you reduce the amount of fat in your food, replacing it with safe, low calorie, nutrient-rich plant foods. This will convince your brain that your body is getting all the nutrition it needs.

In fact, you'll be able to eat more food and feel more satisfied while consuming fewer calories and fats.

Plant foods break down slowly in your stomach, making you feel full longer, and they are rich in vitamins, minerals, trace elements, carbohydrates and protein for energy and muscle-building. This allows your body to burn off its excess stored fat.

It's almost impossible to hide from the news and discussion about the obesity epidemic that's taking both lives and shattering the quality of life worldwide. It's in the papers, on television and being blogged about on the internet almost endlessly.

If that's not enough, unless you're blind it's hard to walk the streets of any big city or small town and not see the end product of this epidemic first hand.

The hard brutal truth is that people are getting fatter and fatter and this is a real health crisis that only a fool could ignore.

There are plenty of reasons for this here are just the most blindingly apparent...

Many People Eat Way too Much Way too Often

It's a hard truth that can't be escaped. The human body wasn't designed by nature to eat as much and as often as most people do. This packs on the flabby pounds as our bodies, which are machines that were designed for survival in not so great circumstances are pampered and overfed in a cushy and soft environment. Remove a bit of hunger from our lives and we will pack on fat and pack it on at lightning speed.

A Widespread Avoidance of Exercise

After overeating the next huge issue is under exercising. Having less physical jobs as well as social lives that revolve around the digital rather than the physical once again takes our bodies away from what they were designed for: running, lifting, hunting and playing. The less muscle we carry the lower our metabolism which means even more fat is packed on. Do you see a pattern developing?

Lack of Quality Sleep

The first two obesity builders contribute to the third. Poor diet and lack of exercise offer the fast track to broken sleep patterns which have been shown in more studies than can be counted to also wreck metabolism and pack on fat. Sleepless nights tossing and turning quickly equal an ugly spare tire of flab around the waist.

Medicine and Drugs

Coming along with our increasingly over medicated society are the side effects of all these medications, which commonly include weight gain and lethargy. Cultures who approach health more naturally and holistically have largely avoided this issue and have been also able to avoid the obesity related health concerns that come along with it. Our societies for the most part haven't figured this out yet.

These are just some of the many reasons the obesity plague is spreading in such a quick and deadly manner. There's plenty more, trust me.

The question stands - what can we do about it? How can we turn the tide against obesity?

The answer is, of course, diet and exercise. There's plenty of diverse ideas about both, some good and a few bad.

This guide offers what I feel may be the perfect solution to a vast majority of people's struggle with putting on fat. It's fairly simple and packed with power, in line with both nature and common sense. Most importantly it works and works almost like magic.

It's called the Feast and Famine Diet and it can change your life for the better. After reading this you will be armed with all you need to know about Feast and Famine to make it work and get the lean and healthy body of your dreams.

CHAPTER 1- THE FEAST AND FAMINE DIET-AN OVERVIEW

The Feast and Famine Diet may be new in name, but in practice has been with us for quite some time. It's the latest tweak on an area of diet programs and ideas less commonly referred to as Intermittent Fasting.

Intermittent Fasting is the rage in health, fitness and weight loss circles with its ideas making it to publication and wide practice. It's popular because it works!

Here are the important guiding principles of Feast and Famine, what gives the diet its power. Try not to stray too far from this foundation if you expect to reap the full rewards of Feast and Famine...

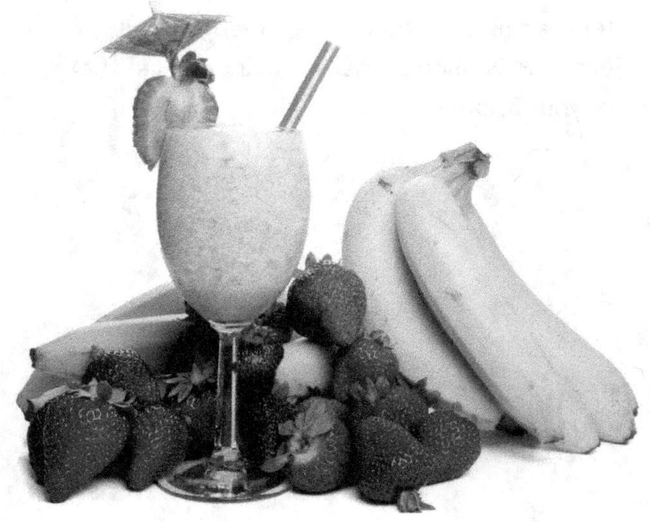

Choose Your Fasting Schedule

There are two approaches generally. The first is alternating Feast days with Famine days, which is personally the method I have seen produce the best weight loss results. The second variant and this is what you will see in intermittent fasting diets like the 5:2 Diet is to eat normally five days and fast two. Our Guide's information works well with both methods, although once again I prefer the first for best long term results as well as ease of use and likelihood of being able to stick with Feast and Famine.

Feasting Guidelines

There's not many. I suggest broadly not eating anything that's junk food or packed with empty calories especially if you are looking to burn off a lot of weight. This will also safeguard your overall health, which is important isn't it? Make sure you get in your fruit and vegetables, but don't be afraid to indulge without binge eating. The fact you have more food freedom at least half the time will make your Famine days much easier to manage psychology.

And succeeding on any diet, Feast and Famine included, is 90% a mental game. In this mental dieting game no diet stacks the deck more in your favor than Feast and

Famine Guidelines

For those needing to drop serious pounds, 500 calories a day on Famine days is a good starting point. This can be adjusted as needed once your weight loss goals are met. Most Feast and Famine enthusiasts like to stay around this area to continue to both reap the health benefits of fasting and to also be able to maintain their Feasting freedom on their Feast days.

* Stay Hydrated. Fasting expert or if you have never fasted in any form before alike, I cannot stress enough the importance of staying hydrated. When your body detoxes on your Famine days and starts to move out some of the junk you have built up, it will go much

smoother if you are drinking a proper amount of water. Ignore this advice and you may just experience some stomach pains, along with the lethargy and weakness that always comes with dehydration regardless of your diet plan.

One of the greatest strengths of intermittent fasting and the Feast and Famine Diet is its simplicity. No diet logs, carbohydrate manipulation schemes and other complications. It works much more dramatically than diets that you need flow charts to follow too. If you can't stick to Feast and Famine it has nothing to do with being confused, but with a lack of will power, self discipline and most of all desire. I think you have those covered, don't you?

CHAPTER 2- GETTING STARTED WITH THE FEAST & FAMINE DIET

Every good idea got its start somewhere. The every other day Feast and Famine Diet has had its way paved for it by earlier intermittent fasting protocols, some a big influence and others not so much, but who still deserve credit for being forward thinkers.

Let's take a look at the history of diets that have come before Feast and Famine and see what we can learn from them. Knowledge is power after all. We have already seen in the mirror and felt in our bodies - that Feast and Famine works big time, we have these pace setters to thank for their experiments and innovations!

First the Warrior

Make no mistake; Ori Hofmekler is certainly a unique guy. Artist, writer and ex-special forces soldier who ran a short lived fitness magazine that was published by a famous Men's magazine company.

During his time as editor in chief he was exposed to the often conflicting ideas of a who's who of dieting gurus of the time, which landed him an obsession with getting to the truth about fat loss.

A few years later came the Warrior Diet book which promotes a 16 hour daily fast followed by a 8 hour eating period. Overall consensus was that it worked, but most people feel the Warrior Diet is difficult to maintain, much more so than every other day fasting ala Feast and Famine. Either way Ori definitely get's credit for the modern birth of intermittent fasting and has served as a great influence on most everyone's ideas who are working with these methods.

Eat Stop Eat

Intermittent Fasting

Eat Stop Eat has been an intermittent fasting dieting method promoted most recently by Brad Pillon. Brad pushes the idea of one or two, zero calorie days a week, the rest of the days eating normally. Once again it's effective and close to what we suggest, but our experience has shown going down to 500 calories every other day is much more effective and manageable than a few days of no calories at all. Not many seem to be able to stick with Eat Stop Eat for long in our experience.

The 5:2 Diet

This is the diet plan most closely related to Feast and Famine and also closest to us on the time line. It's wildly popular in Europe and is gaining ground in places like Hollywood in the USA.

Five days of normal eating followed by two days of reduced calories. Very powerful and all our ideas here work well with the 5:2 Diet. Our opinion holds every other day Feast and Famine is a better fat burner without added psychological tolls. Follow this Guide's advice and I think you will agree!

That's the recent history of intermittent fasting leading us to where we are today. Feast and Famine is the present and I have no doubt it will proudly stand the test of time. It torches fat, is easy to follow, requires really no added expenses in its purest form and promotes over all vibrant health. What's there not to love about Feast and Famine? It's perfect for the health enthusiast who wants to get lean and look great.

CHAPTER 3- THE ADVANTAGES OF THE FEAST & FAMINE DIET

The Feast and Famine Diet brings a load of benefits some more obvious than others. Are you ready to take a look? I think you'll find them really exciting. If radically reducing fat while also basking in these health benefits doesn't interest someone looking to transform their body for the better I'm not sure what will!

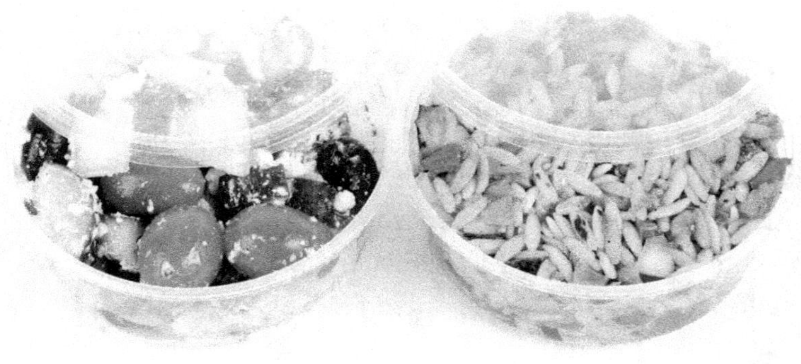

Quickly Cut Body Fat Safely

This is why most people will explore the Feast and Famine approach to diet. You can expect to see the fat melt off as long as you take your Famine days seriously. Eat too much on those days and you are obviously missing the point. We know this works, we've seen it and now even better news - science backs it up!

Recent University of Illinois research has shown in those following alternate day reduced calorie plans (in line with our Guide's recommendations) lost significantly more fat than those eating normally and following the same exercise protocols. It's a plus to be on the right side of science when, sadly, they most often trail far behind the true health and diet vanguard!

Easy To Follow and Manage

The next ground breaking benefit of Feast and Famine is how easy it is to follow and manage. I've touched on this already, but it truly bears repeating. Anyone who has counted carbs on a ketogenic diet like Atkins or the many others I'm sure will quickly agree! Once you figure out in your head what your 500 or 600 calories on famine days looks like you are set. No calculators or complications, period.

Enhanced Mental Function

Yes, we suspected it, but science has backed us up again. Reduced weekly calories (which is what you get with the

 Feast and Famine Diet) leads to increased focus, better memory and other enhanced cognitive function according to Mark Mattson's research for the Lancet. These effects may even carry over into the fight against Alzheimer's disease and other similar huge health concerns which Mattson is exploring further.

Improve Insulin Levels

One of the reasons why many people pack on and find it so hard to lose body fat is their out of whack insulin levels. The Feast and Famine approach optimizes insulin levels for healthy fat loss, which just adds to the amount of fat already being cut from the calorie reduction and heightened metabolism we've already touched on.

Frees Up Time on Famine Days

One of the surprise benefits of this approach is the new found time you find available on Famine days. Small meals and no constant snacking or grazing frees up a shocking amount of time and energy that can be used positively elsewhere. I've found, and others have confirmed this, that some of our most creative and productive days turn out again and again to be famine days! Far from not having energy you end up filled with it!

The Feast and Famine Diet approach is packed with benefits, physical, mental and even social. It's hard to even think of anything, but a small drawback or two and then only for those who are lacking in the desire to "get lean" department. This is truly a method that changes lives for the best.

CHAPTER 4- HOW TO PREPARE FOR THE FAST

Any diet requires a bit of preparation at first, Feast and Famine is certainly not an exception. I will say it requires much less preparation by the nature of Feast and Famine than any other diet I can think of and you won't have to jump many hurdles, do any real expensive shopping or experience any of the other more traditional diet headaches.

Here are some tips to get ready to get the most out our plan...

If Possible At First Food Shop More Often

Here's a trick I used in the beginning days of my intermittent fasting experiments and I've suggested to many of my friends and clients who have given it high praise too. Only keep enough food on hand for the days needs. On Feasting days you will have the pleasure of picking out some new treat to indulge in and on Famine days you won't be as tempted to cheat as you would be if the refrigerator is packed with snacks. Now if you live rurally, or have a large family this may be less practical, but if you can do it I guarantee it will give you a big advantage over those who ignore this tip.

If You Skip A Day Just Get Right Back On Schedule

This diet is about freedom and abundance not restriction. If you have a family event, a date or even a slight slip up on a Famine day just get right back in action the next day and reduce your calories. No master dietary equations are fouled or other nonsense. Now don't make a habit of this or you may end up seeing less than optimal results, but once in a while is perfectly fine. This automatic leeway is built into the Feast and Famine program making it not a diet you can "fail" at if you stumble while getting into the groove, or any other time really!

Throw Out Your Past Diet Experiences

Feast and Famine requires a whole new view of dieting, so in all likelihood your past dieting experiences positive and especially negative don't offer a whole lot of relevance. I'd suggest you file them away and don't let them influence what you are doing here and now. This attitude, not only in dieting and fitness, but also in other areas of life can break chains and open up doors. See what you think.

Are you feeling more ready to begin? You should be because there's a bright, fit and happy new you waiting at the end of the Feast and Famine road. And it's a road not particularly long in most cases or even exceedingly difficult. You've taken the first step by reading this Guide, don't turn back now!

CHAPTER 5- TYPICAL MISTAKES BEGINNERS MAKE

Now just because the Feast and Famine Diet is easy to understand and simple to apply to your lifestyle doesn't mean it's easy for all to practice or it's impossible to make mistakes. In fact some mistakes with intermittent fasting are fairly common among beginners, let's go over them and see if you can't avoid these pitfalls before you make them rather than after. A few of these I even learned the hard way!

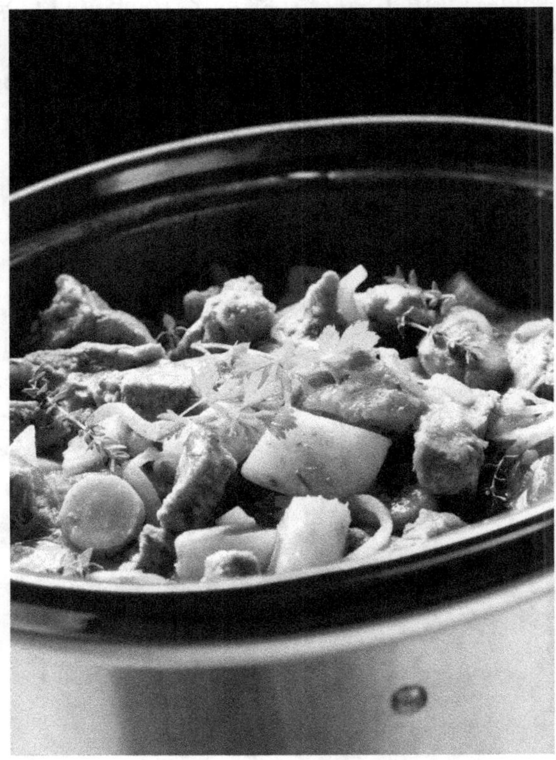

Pigging Out on Too Much on Junk Food

Let's be serious for a second on the subject of getting lean and healthy. While we are allowed and encouraged to eat loosely and enjoyably on Feast days this doesn't mean we have a license to eat completely like a glutton. So if you are not losing weight the way you'd like to be and are eating endless chips, ice cream and candy on your Feast days tighten up your diet and eat healthier.

You should be striving to optimize your health anyway shouldn't you?

Being Scared to Death of Hunger

No one has ever starved to death eating 500 calories or less every other day. Nor have they damaged their body in any way. So if you are experiencing great stress and discomfort over being hungry every other day, it's time to gain more control over your mind. This is done by developing your will power doing things like following this diet even when you would rather not be, focusing on your desired end result. Be tough and be rewarded.

Eating Too Much On Famine Days

Let's not play games, 500 calories or less means 500 calories or less. If you are eating clean on your Feast days and still not losing weight it likely means you are eating too much on Famine days. Cut down what you are eating and if you must check the calorie counts to make sure you are at 500 calories or under.

Reducing Your Level of Activity

It's tempting for some to slow down their activities on Famine days. Don't fall into this. In fact with a little Feast and Famine experience under your belt you will realize Famine days actually free up more energy and you should strive to be even more active. Doing more is almost always better than doing nothing as long as you can do it safely.

Putting Yourself Unnecessarily Around People Who Don't Respect Your Diet Efforts.

Apart from close friends and family who it would be difficult to avoid, it's a downer to be around people who try to talk negatively about or discourage you from meeting your Feast and Famine goals. Again dieting is 90% mental so don't let other people mess with your mental game. It's annoying, defeatist and unnecessary!

These common beginner mistakes are all easy to avoid and if you stumble it's ok just keep going. The Feast and Famine Diet has been designed to be both effective, open and user friendly. A little bit of self-reflection and you are quickly back on course and seizing the body and life of your dreams!

CHAPTER 6- FEAST DAY SAMPLE MENU

The Feast and Famine Feast Day! Now comes the fun part, my friends! Let's dig deep into a sample Feast day while we are following the Feast and Famine Diet.

This is taken from my own lifestyle and from a period of time when I was consistently losing weight as fast as I ever had every week without fail. My metabolism has never been superhuman either, so rest assured if this has worked for me it's very, very likely to work for you as well (with portion sizes adjusted if you are female, of course.)

Read on and enjoy. I hope it gets you filled with enthusiasm! You will notice I'm not including calories, because who counts calories on a Feast day?! I sure don't and you shouldn't either.

Breakfast

Breakfast is regarded by many nutrition experts as being the most important meal of the day. It's also a meal I've neglected most of my life due to the perils of enjoying sleeping in. Intermittent fasting has cleared that up - after a 500 calorie day I can't wait to really eat a substantial breakfast! I must say I feel much more ready for action after a full force breakfast.

4 Eggs Scrambled. I choose to go with whole eggs for hormonal optimization's sake, but often mix up the ways the eggs are prepared.

Fresh Tomato, Onion and Jalapeno Salsa. Extra hot and used as a condiment on top of my eggs.

4 pieces of Turkey Bacon. I will eat other styles of bacon when turkey bacon isn't available.

Intermittent Fasting

4oz of Steak Sauteed in Frying Pan. I only add this when I really want to indulge or if I feel like I need the extra protein for muscle building purposes.

8oz Milk. Whole milk is also great for guys looking to naturally boost their hormonal advantage,

Snack

A few handfuls of Organic Almonds

Small Spinach Salad. I don't use dressing beyond olive oil and garlic and sometimes toss in some tomatoes, onion and cucumber depending what's on hand.

Lunch

Medium Baked Potato. I dress the potato with a bit of butter and garlic.

Two 6oz Grilled Chicken Breasts. Sometimes plain or sometimes with salsa on top if I have extra from breakfast.

Small Side of Mixed Vegetables. Snack

More Almonds!

Dinner

10oz Grilled Lean Steak. Plain beyond salt and pepper.

Small side salad or spinach salad. Side Portion of White or Brown Rice.

As much Green Tea as I'd like to drink sweetened with pure stevia.

Occasionally a desert of organic sorbet, a small addiction of mine!

Snack

Stacie Williams
My after dinner snack is pretty wide open within reason. If I eat chips I make sure to not go overboard.

Vanilla Whey Protein shake made with half whole milk and half almond milk. I drink this right before bed.

This is just a sample Feast and Famine Feast day, but it should give you a great idea of what's possible when we eat smartly and abundantly. The real eye opener is when you eat like this half the time and still see the fat melting away. That's when you will become a full force Feast and Famine true believer!

CHAPTER 7- FAMINE DAY SAMPLE MENU

Now after seeing a sample Feast and Famine Feast day it's time for a sample of the flip side - the all important Famine day where we will fast eating vastly reduced calories activating our metabolism, our "skinny gene" and setting ourselves up for both body transformation and all the other health benefits we have already discussed. This is again, from my own personal experience and the daily calorie total is focused on the magic number of 500 calories. I think you will find this a very manageable day that will hardly leave you suffering.

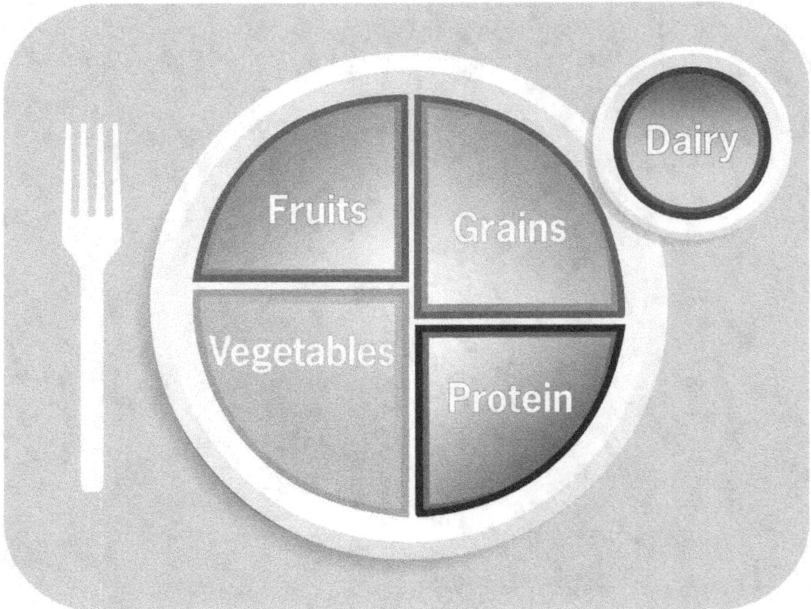

Pre-Breakfast

16oz Spring Water immediately upon wakening.

A cup of Fresh Coffee, no milk or cream sweetened with stevia. 0 calories.

Breakfast

A second cup of Fresh Coffee, no milk or cream sweetened with Stevia. 0 calories.

8oz Spring Water.

Now this doesn't seem like much of a breakfast, but I prefer to sleep in a bit and save my calories for lunch and dinner. This is my own personal choice and you may choose to distribute your calories differently if you are more of a morning person!

Snack

8oz Green Tea sweetened with stevia. 0 calories.

12oz Spring water. Lunch

Finally time to get in some food, paying special intention

NOT to overdo it. This is the meal when many feel most tempted, since while eating a small dinner you know a large breakfast is coming up relatively quickly. Don't give in!

Two medium hard boiled eggs. Once again I like to make sure I eat whole eggs every day to maximize my hormonal optimization plan. You have the option of egg whites, egg beaters and so on. 175

Calories.

Two slices Whole Wheat Toast. Sometimes I eat the eggs on the toast and sometimes as a side depending on mood. 115 Calories.

A cup of Fresh Coffee, no milk or cream sweetened with stevia. 0 calories.

8oz spring water.

Total Lunch calories: 290 give or take.

Snack

8oz Green Tea sweetened with Stevia. 0 calories. Yes, I do love caffeine on Famine day in case you were wondering. It serves to boost energy, raise metabolism and even acts as a mild appetite suppressant.

12oz Spring water. Dinner

Half a cup (after cooked) Spaghetti with a small amount of low fat / low calorie butter, salt, pepper and garlic. 150 calories.

One slice whole wheat toast. 55 calories.

12oz Spring Water.

Total calorie intake for the day roughly 495 calories. This puts right where we are hoping to be on a Famine day. I repeat these meals often since they are pretty much decision free and simple to prepare. They can also easily be ordered in all but the most incompetent of restaurants!

One last bit of advice - take a half hour on Sunday and figure out your five hundred calorie and below meals for the week rather than just trying to wing it and guess how many calories you are eating on Famine days on the fly.

This will end up equating in much more weight loss over the long term and also save you a few headaches and a bit of possible confusion too. When in doubt repeat meals! Don't worry about getting bored a Feast day is less than 24 hours away!

CHAPTER 8- HOW TO SHOP

Now that we hopefully have agreed that the Feast and Famine Diet is more than do-able after looking at a sample Feast day and a sample Famine day I thought I'd share with you a few more intermittent fasting insider's secrets.

The fine art of shopping while following Feast and Famine. Although all of us develop our style of eating while on the diet which best suits our individual needs I've found having an experience veteran's shopping list can provide some helpful guidelines. So are you ready to go shopping Feast and Famine style? Let's do it!

Here's what we are packing our shopping cart with...

Non-hormonal Chicken Breasts. I'm a bit of a chicken addict and don't think I could live without it. I eat chicken at least once a day on Feast days, sometimes twice. I think of chicken as a sort of "neutral" protein that can be prepared in so many ways it's wise to fall in love with.

Make sure the fat is trimmed off!

Non-hormonal Grass Fed Lean Beef. Another Feast day favorite, especially when I'm hitting it more heavily in the gym. When you are looking to put on muscle while cutting fat on Feast and Famine aim for around 1 gram of protein for every pound you weigh.

Eggs. As you've seen eggs are on the meal agenda often for both Feast and Famine days. Don't skip them, unless you are one of the few who can't stomach the thought of them!

A variety of Pasta. Organic Spinach

Organic Leaf Lettuce. I should add organic produce is not a must, but I try to stick with it when I can.

Tomatoes.

Onions.

Miso soup. Miso soup is great for a change of pace on Famine days and has been shown in research to have all sorts of regenerative and health boosting qualities. Plus it tastes great too!

Green Tea. Essential. Green Tea is great for a extra fat burning boost, is inexpensive and calorie free.

Coffee. Spring Water.

Whey Protein. I've tried to avoid any supplement recommendations as the Feast and Famine Diet works great without them, but a good protein shake is the one exception. Keep your protein levels high and you will have no worries at all about losing muscle while cutting body fat.

Stevia. A all natural and calorie free sweetener which will make you forget sugar ever even existed. A true gift from above.

Almonds. A go to snack.

Now a look at this list reveals that avoiding overly processed and junk food isn't a bad idea and you can still really Feast without it. That way if you go a bit crazy at a friend's or eating out occasionally your body won't even notice it. Buying too many terrible food choices probably sends the wrong message to your subconscious and may set up many for binge eating and failure. Some intermittent fasting experts disagree, but this is what my own personal experience has revealed. After you move beyond the beginner stage feel free to experiment!

CHAPTER 9- INCORPORATING THE FEAST & FAMINE DIET INTO YOUR LIFESTYLE

The only way to really lose weight and keep it off is to make the mental switch from thinking in terms of short term dieting to the more dynamic perspective of making lasting healthy lifestyle choices.

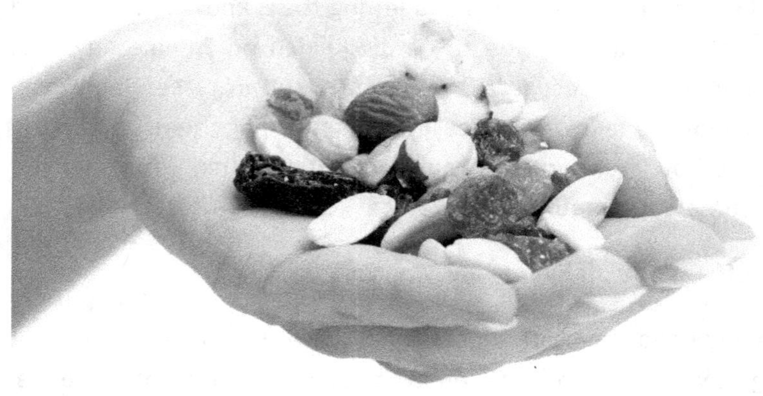

Feast and Famine is the perfect tool to help you make that change. In fact after studying and experimenting with every major diet of the last decade, I can honestly say none in my opinion are better suited for a long term lifestyle choice than intermittent fasting and Feast and Famine. It's easy to manage, inexpensive to follow, relatively pleasant and enjoyable and very, very powerful. This covers nearly every category of a dream long term eating plan check list I can think of!

Here are some tips in incorporating Feast and Famine into your lifestyle

Celebrate Your Successes with Feast and Famine

Thinking positive and choosing to focus on the positive changes you have made while intermittent fasting will go a long way in solidifying it as a part of your lasting lifestyle. Try your best to not dwell on any poor weeks or bumps in the road you may experience. This will pay off huge dividends both in weight loss and in life. Again 90% of the game is mental, let's not forget.

Recruit Those Closest To You to Lend a Hand

Making your significant other close friends and family aware of how Feast and Famine works and letting them know you could use their help encouraging you to be disciplined on Famine days will help this healthy lifestyle really cement itself in place. Some may even choose to take up the Feast and Famine flag themselves when they see how great you look and feel. That's when you know you are really onto something!

Take off a Week off Every Few Months

Everyone needs a vacation occasionally. This will prevent burn out and give yourself a great pat on the back after months of discipline. If you can time your vacation from Feast and Famine with a real vacation from work or school even better! I've found a week off really helps recharge enthusiasm's batteries and allow me to plunge back into the Feast and Famine lifestyle full force.

Keep Expanding Your Knowledge of Intermittent Fasting

A final way to make sure you stick with Feast and Famine as a lifestyle choice is to keep your brain engaged in learning new knowledge about intermittent fasting in all its forms. Join some forums, follow the news and the blogs and if you go to a gym make friends with others living this way of life. This will continually confirm what you are doing is both healthy and a good choice. It's always a good idea to have as big a support circle as possible.

Stacie Williams

Even if you take up Feast and Famine to lose some weight quickly planning to go back to your old ways of eating, let me warn you, you may very well end up hooked and sticking around for the duration. The good news is your body will be much healthier and look much better for your efforts. Breaking from the norm into a lifestyle that gets the most out of body and mind is a benefit that's priceless. Embrace it!

CHAPTER 10- FAT BURNING FOOD TIPS

Each one of the following foods is clinically proven to promote weight loss. These foods go a step beyond simply adding no fat to your system – they possess special properties that add zip to your system and help your body melt away unhealthy pounds. These incredible foods can suppress your appetite for junk food and keep your body running smoothly with clean fuel and efficient energy.

You can include these foods in any sensible weight-loss plan. They give your body the extra metabolic kick that it needs to shave off weight quickly.

A sensible weight loss plan calls for no fewer than 1,200 calories per day. But Dr. Charles Klein recommends consuming more than that, if you can believe it – 1,500 to 1,800 calories per day. He says you will still lose weight quite effectively at that intake level without endangering your health.

Hunger is satisfied more completely by filling the stomach. Ounce for ounce, the foods listed below accomplish that better than any others. At the same time, they're rich in nutrients and possess special fat-melting talents.

Apples

These marvels of nature deserve their reputation for keeping the doctor away when you eat one a day. And now, it seems, they can help you melt the fat away, too.

First of all, they elevate your blood glucose (sugar) levels in a safe, gentle manner and keep them up longer than most foods. The practical effect of this is to leave you feeling satisfied longer, say researchers.

Secondly, they're one of the richest sources of soluble fiber in the supermarket. This type of fiber prevents hunger pangs by guarding against dangerous swings or drops in your blood sugar level, says Dr. James Anderson of the University of Kentucky's School of Medicine.

An average size apple provides only 81 calories and has no sodium, saturated fat or cholesterol. You'll also get the added health benefits of lowering the level of cholesterol already in your blood as well as lowering your blood pressure.

Whole Grain Bread

You needn't dread bread. It's the butter, margarine or cream cheese you put on it that's fattening, not the bread itself. We'll say this as often as needed – fat is fattening. If you don't believe that, ponder this – a gram of carbohydrate has four calories, a gram of protein four, and a gram of fat nine. So which of these is really fattening?

Bread, a natural source of fiber and complex carbohydrates, is okay for dieting. Norwegian scientist Dr. Bjarne Jacobsen found that people who eat less than two slices of bread daily weigh about 11 pounds more that those who eat a lot of bread.

Studies at Michigan State University show some bread actually reduce the appetite.

Researchers compared white bread to dark, high-fiber bread and found that students who ate 12 slices a day of the dark, high-fiber bread felt less hunger on a daily basis and lost five pounds in two months. Others who ate white bread were hungrier, ate more fattening foods and lost no weight during this time.

So the key is eating dark, rich, high-fiber breads such as pumpernickel, whole wheat, mixed grain, oatmeal and others. The average slice of whole grain bread contains only 60 to 70 calories,

Intermittent Fasting
is rich in complex carbohydrates – the best, steadiest fuel you can give your body – and delivers surprising amount of protein.

Coffee

Easy does it is the password here. We've all heard about potential dangers of caffeine – including anxiety and insomnia – so moderation is the key.

The caffeine in coffee can speed up the metabolism. In nutritional circles, it's known as a metabolic enhancer, according to Dr. Judith Stern of the University of California at Davis.

This makes sense, since caffeine is a stimulant. Studies show it can help you burn more calories than normal, perhaps up to 10 percent more. For safety's sake, it's best to limit your intake to a single cup in the morning and one in the afternoon. Add only skim milk to tit and try doing without sugar – many people learn to love it that way.

Grapefruit

There's good reason for this traditional diet food to be a regular part of your diet. It helps dissolve fat and cholesterol, according to Dr. James Cerd of the University of Florida. An average sized grapefruit has 74 calories, delivers a whopping 15 grams of pectin (the special fiber linked to lowering cholesterol and fat), is high in vitamin C and potassium and is free of fat and sodium.

It's rich in natural galacturonic acid, which adds to its potency as a fat and cholesterol fighter. The additional benefit here is assistance in the battle against atherosclerosis (hardening of the arteries) and the development of heart disease. Try sprinkling it with cinnamon rather than sugar to take away some of the tart taste.

Mustard

Try the hot, spicy kind you find in Asian import stores, specialty shops and exotic groceries. Dr. Jaya Henry of Oxford Polytechnic Institute in England, found that the amount of hot mustard normally called for in Mexican, Indian and Asian recipes, about one teaspoon, temporarily speeds up the metabolism, just as caffeine and the drug ephedrine do.

"But mustard is natural and totally safe," Henry says. "It can be used every day, and it really works. I was shocked to discover it can speed up the metabolism by as much as 20 to 25 percent for several hours." This can result in the body burning an extra 45 calories for every 700 consumed, Dr. Henry says.

Peppers

Hot, spicy chili peppers fall into the same category as hot mustard, Henry says. He studied them under the same circumstances as the mustard and they worked just as well. A mere three grams of chili peppers were added to a meal consisting of 766 total calories. The peppers' metabolism-raising properties worked like a charm, leading to what Henry calls a diet-induced thermic effect. It doesn't take much to create the effect. Most salsa recipes call for four to eight chilies – that's not a lot.

Peppers are astonishingly rich in vitamins A and C, abundant in calcium, phosphorus, iron and magnesium, high in fiber, free of fat, low in sodium and have just 24 calories per cup.

Potatoes

We've got to be kidding, right? Wrong. Potatoes have developed the same "fattening" rap as bread, and it's unfair. Dr. John McDougal, director of the nutritional medicine clinic at St. Helena Hospital in Deer Park, California, says, "An excellent food with which to achieve rapid weight loss is the potato, at 0.6 calories per gram or about 85 calories per potato." A great source of fiber and potassium, they lower cholesterol and protect against strokes and heart disease.

Preparation and toppings are crucial. Steer clear of butter, milk and sour cream, or you'll blow it. Opt for yogurt instead.

Rice

An entire weight-loss plan, simple called the Rice Diet, was developed by Dr. William Kempner at Duke University in Durham, North Carolina. The diet, dating to the 1930's, makes rice the staple of your food intake. Later on, you gradually mix in various fruits and vegetables.

It produces stunning weight loss and medical results. The diet has been shown to reverse and cure kidney ailments and high blood pressure.

A cup of cooked rice (150 grams) contains about 178 calories — approximately one-third the number of calories found in an equivalent amount of beef or cheese. And remember, whole grain rice is much better for you than white rice.

Soups

Soup is good for you! Maybe not the canned varieties from the store — but old-fashioned, homemade soup promotes weight loss. A study by Dr. John Foreyt of Baylor College of Medicine in Houston, Texas, found that dieters who ate a bowl of soup before lunch and dinner lost more weight than dieters who didn't. In fact, the more soup they ate, the more weight they lost. And soup eaters tend to keep the weight off longer.

Naturally, the type of soup you eat makes a difference. Cream soups or those made of beef or pork are not your best bets. But here's a great recipe:

Stacie Williams

Slice three large onions, three carrots, four stalks of celery, one zucchini and one yellow squash. Place in a kettle. Add three cans crushed tomatoes, two packets low-sodium chicken bouillon, three cans water and one cup white wine (optional). Add tarragon, basil, oregano, thyme and garlic powder. Boil, then simmer for an hour. Serves six.

Spinach

Popeye really knew what he was talking about, according to Dr. Richard Shekelle, an epidemiologist at the University of Texas. Spinach has the ability to lower cholesterol, rev up the metabolism and burn away fat. Rich in iron, beta carotene and vitamins C and E, it supplies most of the nutrients you need.

Tofu

You just can't say enough about this health food from Asia. Also called soybean curd, it's basically tasteless, so any spice or flavoring you add blends with it nicely. A 2½ " square has 86 calories and nine grams of protein. (Experts suggest an intake of about 40 grams per day.) Tofu contains calcium and iron, almost no sodium and not a bit of saturated fat. It makes your metabolism run on high and even lowers cholesterol. With different varieties available, the firmer tofus are goof for stir-frying or adding to soups and sauces while the softer ones are good for mashing, chopping and adding to salads.

CHAPTER 11- CONCLUSION

Thanks for taking the time to read our Guide and I truly hope you have found it helpful and eye opening. I have no doubt if you throw your focus into the Feast and Famine Diet you will achieve your weight loss goals and much more.

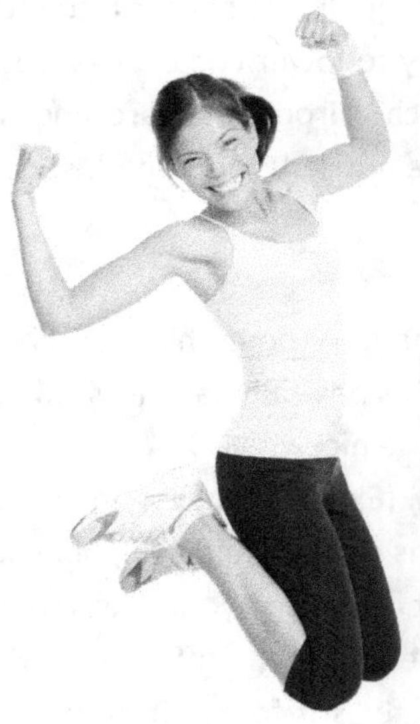

That said when do you plan to start? If you just hesitated you may be experiencing the greatest foe of achieving the body of your dreams of them all - the evil called procrastination. Before I leave let me share with you some tips that can help you slay that beast and begin your own transformation story today!

Just Do It

The Feast and Famine Diet requires no special food, no supplements and no information, really, beyond this Guide to work and work well. So what are you waiting for? Start Feast and Famine right NOW. The only thing stopping you is your own inertia. Banish any thoughts of tomorrow or next week. Once again make a decision and start NOW.

Expose Your Excuses

Do you have reoccurring excuses why you can't start intermittent fasting today? Say these excuses out loud so you can hear how ridiculously self defeating they are. If you are still in doubt write them down and burn them as you free yourself from limiting beliefs.

Look At Yourself Naked In The Mirror.

If you are fat the mirror and a lack of clothes won't lie. Remind yourself your body won't change into something more pleasing until you first make a decision to change it and then second move forward with action in support of that decision. That action is to wisely adopt the Feast and Famine Diet. If not you will likely look the same, if not worse, than you did in the mirror in the days, weeks, months and years to come. This may sound harsh, but a harsh truth is much better than a pleasant falsehood.

Quit Time Wasters

Do you need so much social media, television or playing video games when your body isn't where you desire it to be? Are you putting the easy and distracting before the vital and important? If so why? Break the trance, quit the time wasters and build the new you NOW!

Write Goals Down As Clearly and Detailed As Possible

Intermittent Fasting

There's a certain magic about the written word, especially when it comes to setting and achieving goals. This magic is even more pronounced when the written words are your own. Write down your goals big and small, read them and embrace Feast and Famine as a means to carry you in the direction you need to be headed. There isn't a success coach or sports psychologist alive who would argue against that advice! You shouldn't either.

Are you psyched about moving forward with Feast and Famine? I knew you would be. This could be a day you look back on decades from now and say "that's where I committed to serious life enhancing change!" The things offered by this lifestyle are just that serious. I'd love to hear your success story so please stay strong and in touch!

ABOUT THE AUTHOR

Stacie Williams has tried her fair share of diets in a bid to lose weight,. What she has found is that a lot of them really only work for the short term. When she was about o give up she was introduced to intermittent fasting. She found it a bit strange and thought that she would be more prone to eat more when the period of fasting was over. She tried it and found that it was the solution that she was looking for.

Now she spends her time teaching others about intermittent fasting. It is a much better option in her opinion than many of the fad diets out there.

Keeping Emotions in Check

A No-Boundaries Guide to Anger Management

By: Kimberly Harris

9781635012750

PUBLISHERS NOTES
Disclaimer – Speedy Publishing LLC

This publication is intended to provide helpful and informative material. It is not intended to diagnose, treat, cure, or prevent any health problem or condition, nor is intended to replace the advice of a physician. No action should be taken solely on the contents of this book. Always consult your physician or qualified health-care professional on any matters regarding your health and before adopting any suggestions in this book or drawing inferences from it.

The author and publisher specifically disclaim all responsibility for any liability, loss or risk, personal or otherwise, which is incurred as a consequence, directly or indirectly, from the use or application of any contents of this book.

Any and all product names referenced within this book are the trademarks of their respective owners. None of these owners have sponsored, authorized, endorsed, or approved this book.

Always read all information provided by the manufacturers' product labels before using their products. The author and publisher are not responsible for claims made by manufacturers.

This book was originally printed before 2014. This is an adapted reprint by Speedy Publishing LLC with newly updated content designed to help readers with much more accurate and timely information and data.

Speedy Publishing LLC

40 E Main Street, Newark, Delaware, 19711

Contact Us: 1-888-248-4521

Website: http://www.speedypublishing.co

REPRINTED Paperback Edition: 9781635012750:

Manufactured in the United States of America